The Memes Book

'ASD in Daily Life'

by Alis Rowe

Copyrighted Material

Published by
Lonely Mind Books
London

Copyright © Alis Rowe 2015

First edition 2015

All rights reserved. No part of this publication may be reproduced in any material form (including photocopying or storing it in any medium by electronic means and whether or not transiently or incidentally to some other use of this publication) without written permission of the copyright owner except in accordance with the provisions of the Copyright, Designs and Patents Act 1988 or under the terms of a licence issued by the Copyright Licensing Agency Ltd, 90 Tottenham Court Road, London, England W1T 4LP. Applications for the copyright owner's written permission to reproduce any part of this publication should be addressed to the publisher.

Warning: The doing of an unauthorised act in relation to a copyright work may result in both a civil claim for damages and criminal prosecution.

hello

'The focus of my life is on two things: 1) routine and 2) special interests. I live my life accommodating everything else I have to do, around these two things.'

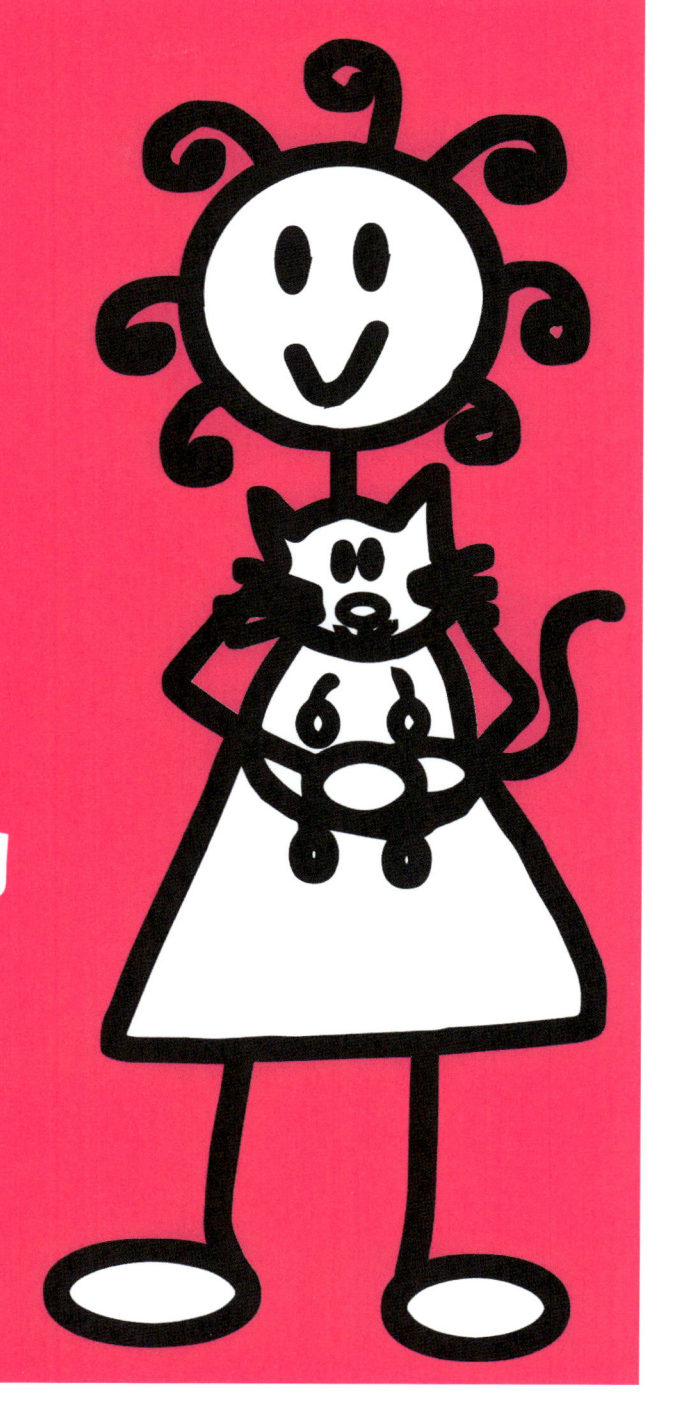

'My favourite days are the days where I can just get on with what I am doing. Days where there are no unexpected social interactions, and I can just focus entirely on what I am doing or what I want to do.'

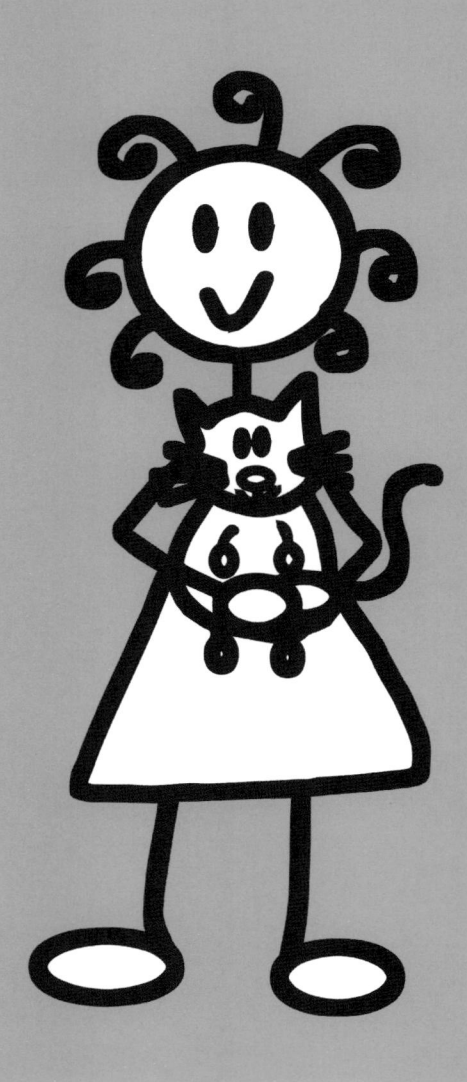

'I always want to be the first one 'in place' before anyone else arrives. I think this is partly because I need to have 'input' drip fed to me, rather than me going from just nothing to a busy, sensory, social too-much-input sort of environment.'

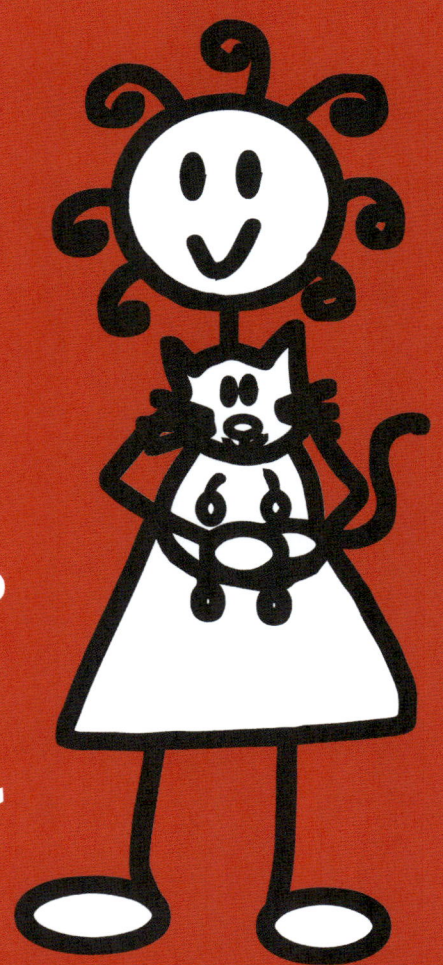

'On the surface, I live a very ordinary life - I have my job and my hobbies and I chat to people at work. But nothing ever really goes beyong the elusive "hello." I just cannot seem to create bonds or make friends.'

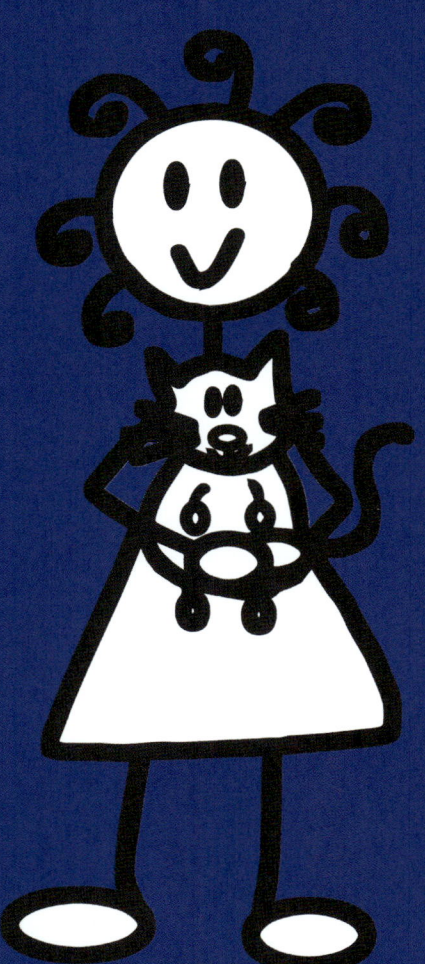

'People with ASD may be prone to getting upset over so called 'trivial' things because, most of the time, even in our 'normal state', we are overwhelmed and confused. When something doesn't quite fit the standard, follow a rule, or have a reason, everything just becomes even more confusing.'

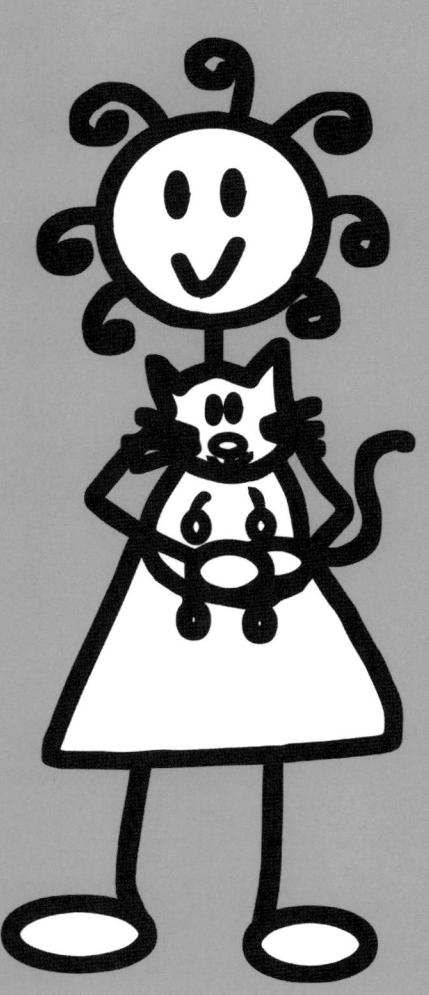

'People stereotype 'disability' as being obvious and severe every time and in every case. But it can also be very subtle and invisible, in the way ASD is.'

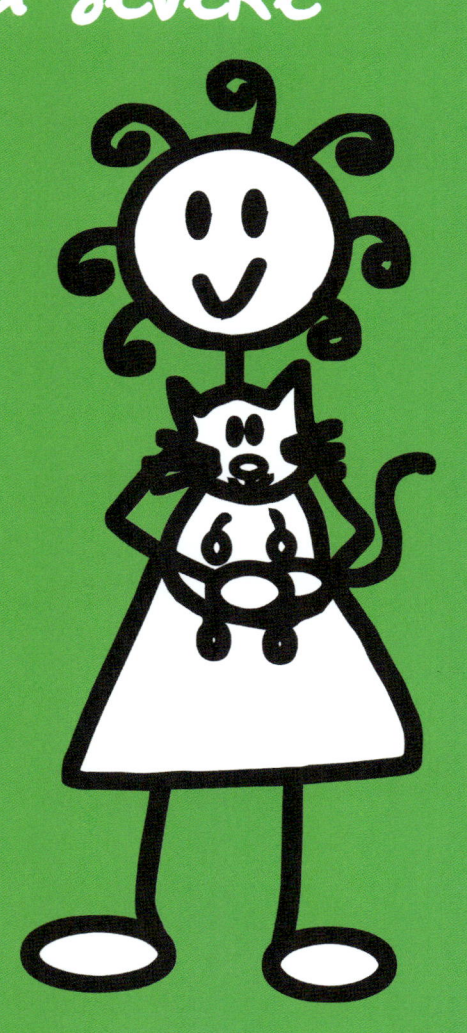

'To have companionship is a basic desire of all human beings. I think this desire is still present in those of us with autism... for introverts it is less. But, regardless, we are challenged by our social communication skills. This paradox causes us to live our lives feeling lonely.'

'We are not always the stereotypical mathematical genii that textbooks about ASD describe, but we may have an extraordinary ability to see patterns in numbers everywhere and lots of us like to count things.'

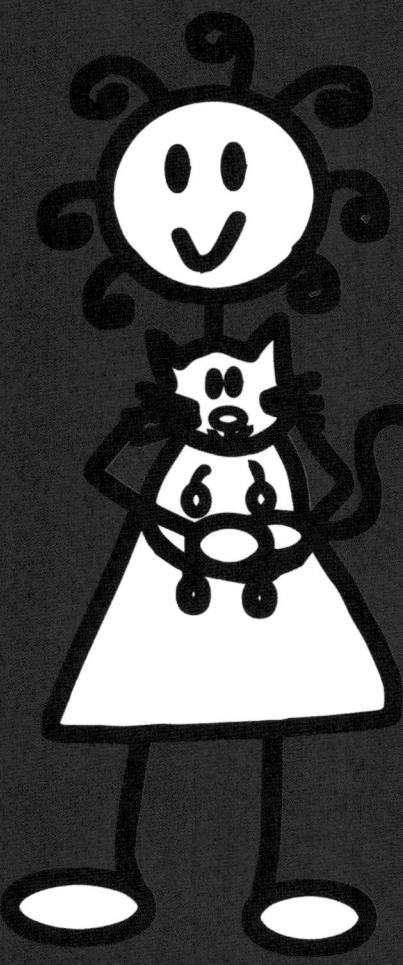

'I don't mind going out and doing 'things' sometimes. However, for me, the pleasure is very short lived and I want to get back home and back to my normal routine as soon as I can.'

'I am a very sentimental person when it comes to familiarity, routines and sameness.'

'I DO NOT LIKE BEING 'FORCED' TO SOCIALISE. I DO NOT LIKE HAVING PRESSURE PUT UPON ME TO BE SOCIAL. I CAN ONLY REALLY COPE WITH SOCIALISING WHEN I AM READY, IN MY OWN TIME.'

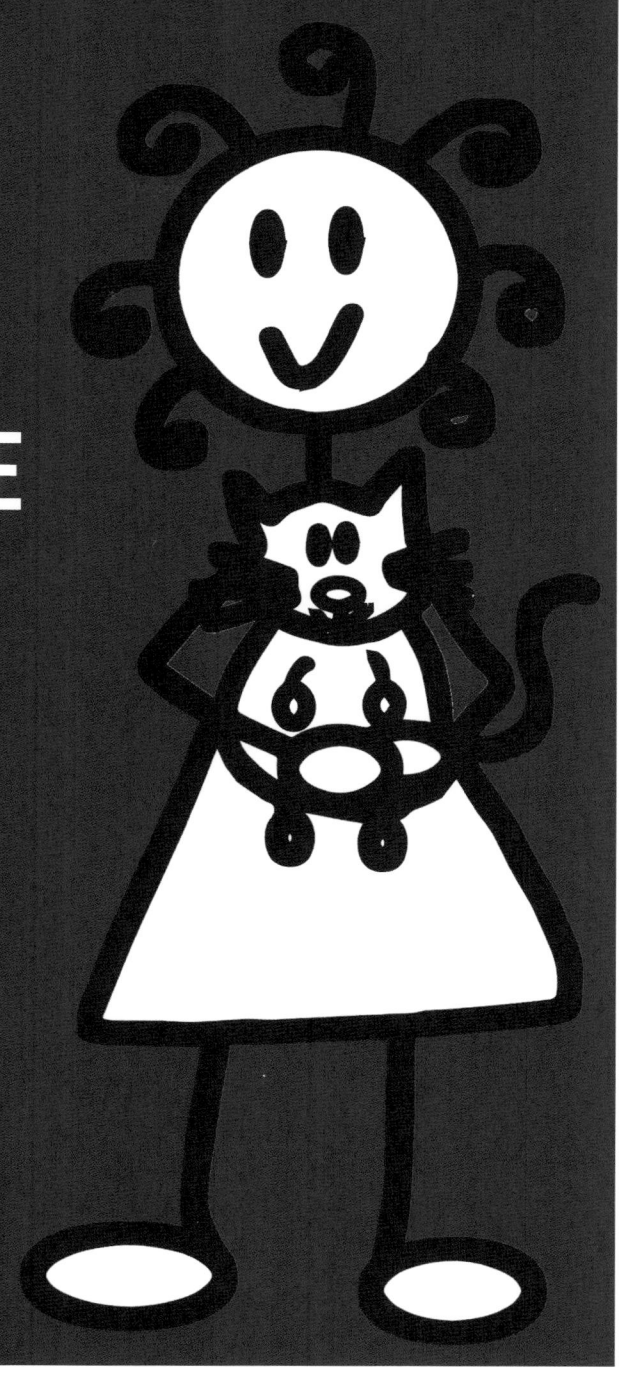

'When I am feeling low, it is easy for me to get consumed in my own worries. I find it helps immensely if I make an extra effort to think about other people and how I can perhaps help them. Being kind and helpful to others, in turn, helps me.'

'When there is a change, it really helps me to learn everything about the change. For example, who caused the change? What is the reason for it? Will things be more efficient because of it? How is it going to affect me?'

"'Big' and 'small' issues are all relative to the person, so no one else should really judge how someone else reacts to something. It is much better to help them solve the issue, no matter how 'big or 'small' it might be.'

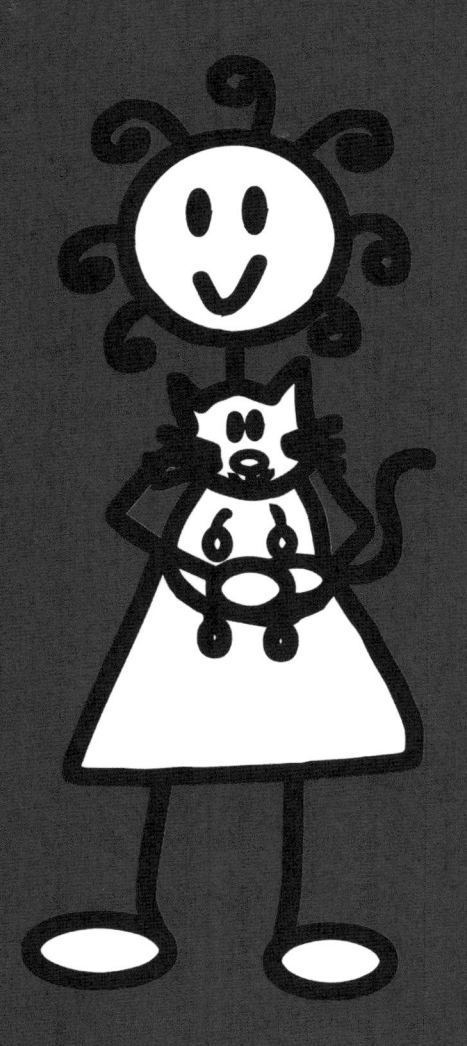

'I want people around me most of the time, but also, most of the time I don't want to chat with them.'

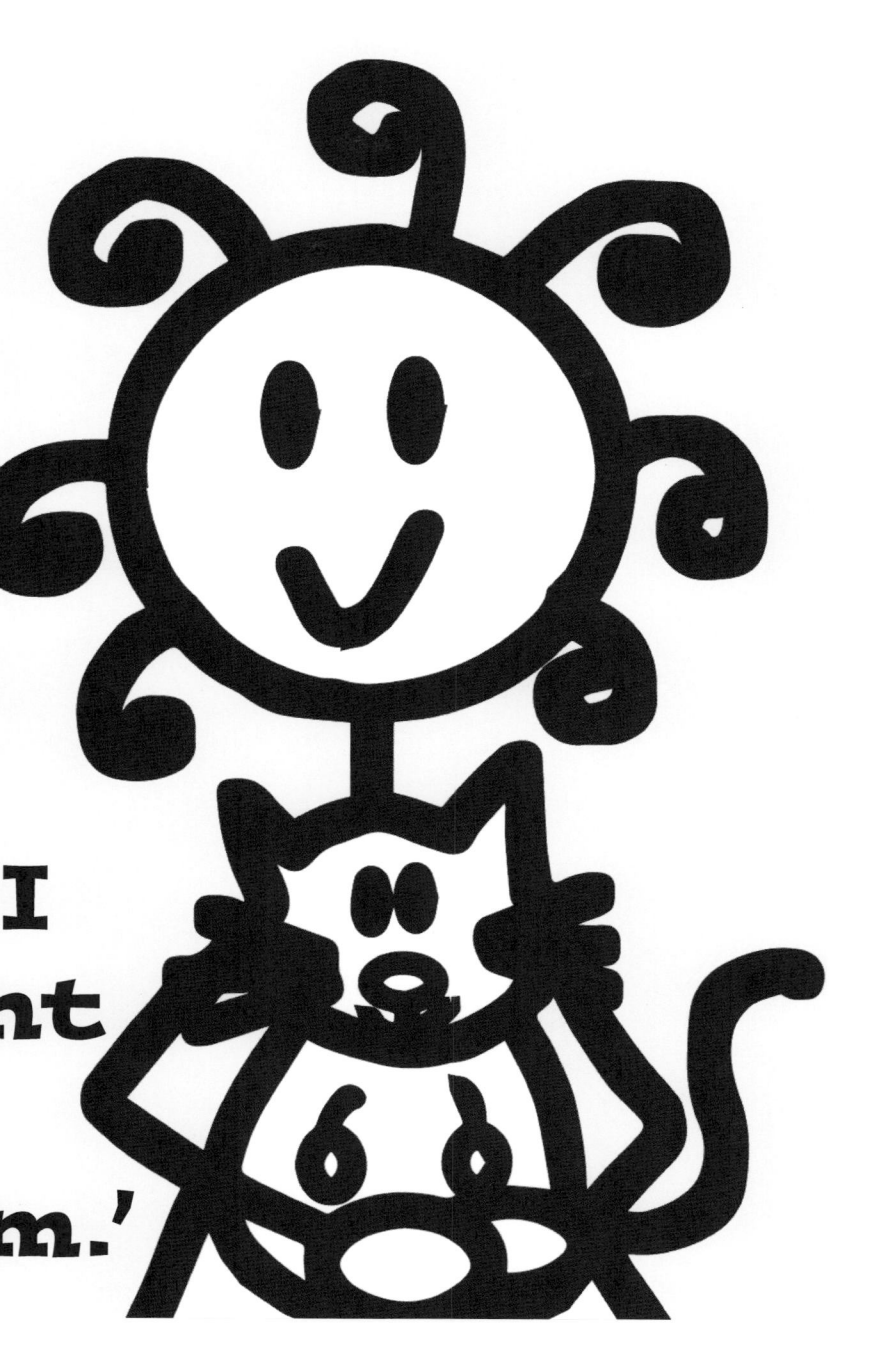

'It is very difficult living a life in which you never know how you're going to 'feel' until the day - not just for yourself but for others as well. It makes planning things incredibly difficult and the last thing you want to do is disrupt or disappoint others.'

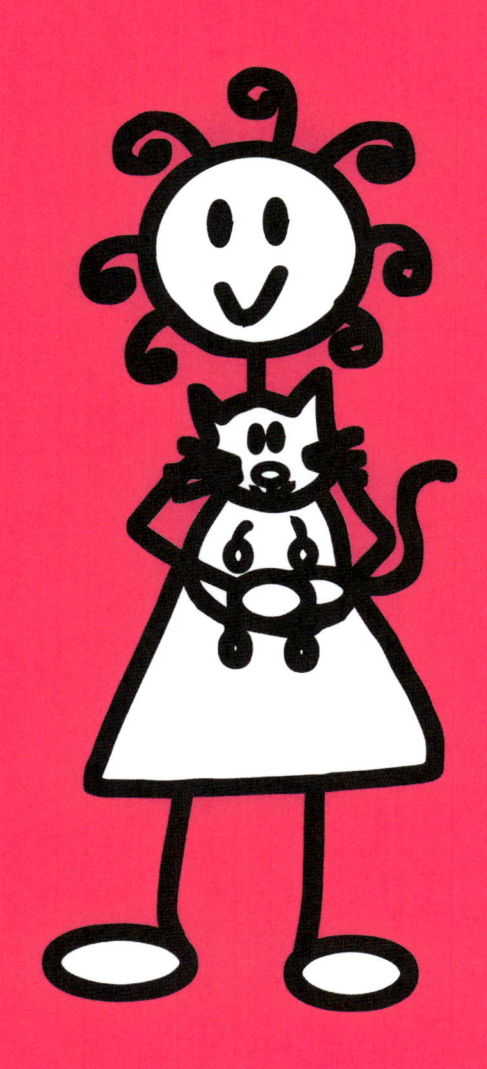

'I don't ever really feel 'present' at social events. I can see everything happening but I'm not able to participate – my mind goes blank and I just feel very, very awkward.'

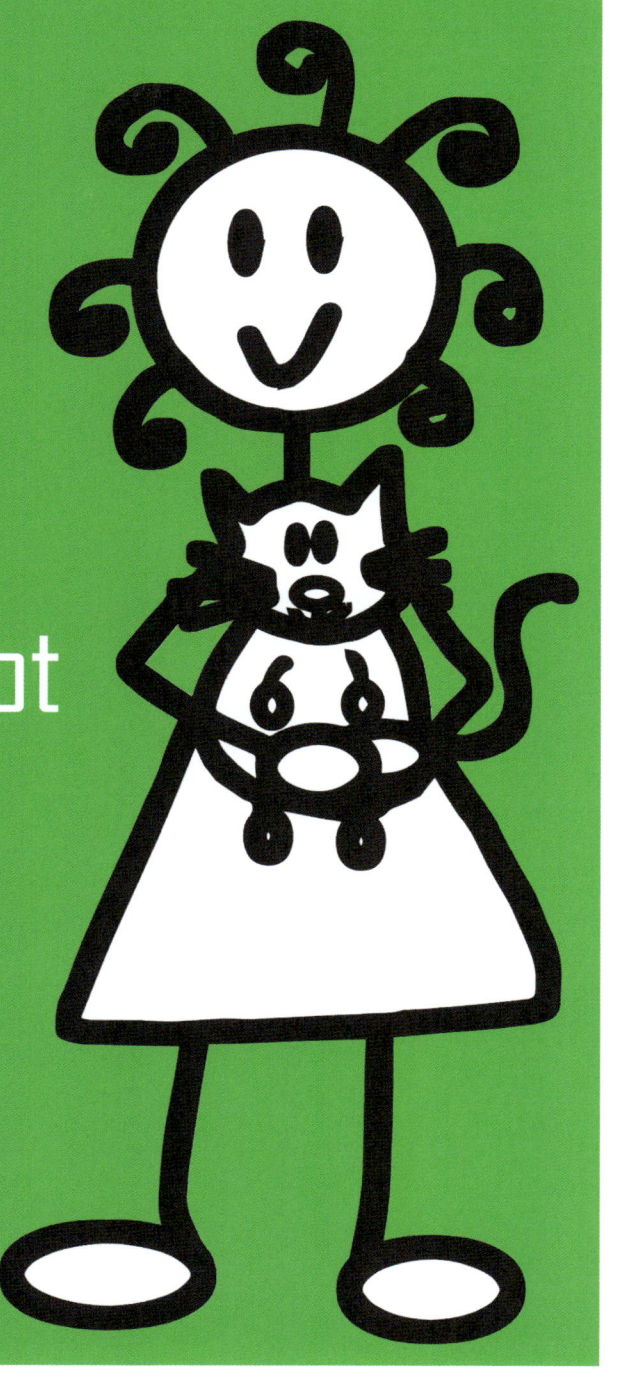

'MY LIFE MAY APPEAR VERY GOOD AND IT CAN APPEAR I AM COPING WELL BUT, UNDERNEATH, MY HAPPINESS IS FRAGILE, AND MY LIFE RESTRICTIVE.'

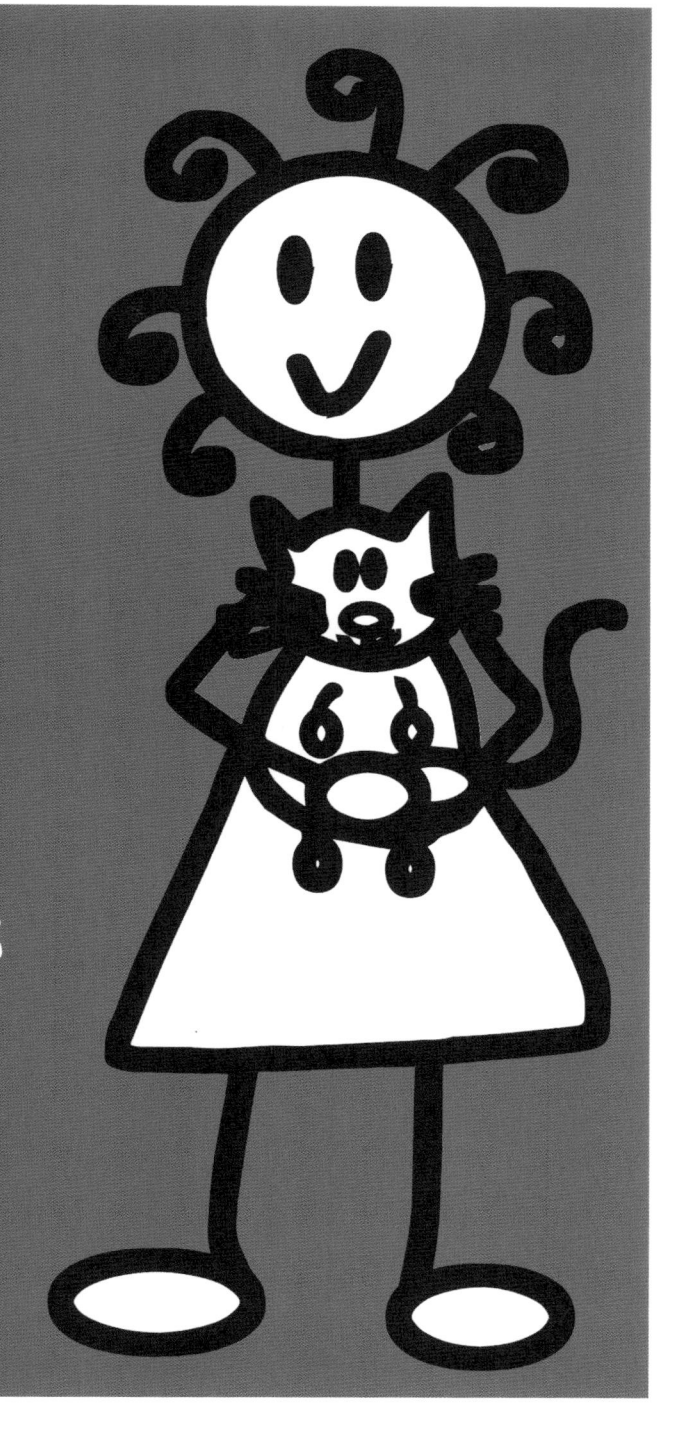

'Generally, when socialising, I end up doing things I don't want to do, just so others feel happy or so that I don't disappoint them.'

'I cope with a lot of situations purely by not being social. It is easier to keep myself to myself.'

'I CAN ONLY FUNCTION AT THE SO CALLED 'HIGH' LEVEL FOR A SMALL AMOUNT OF TIME AND, AFTER THAT AMOUNT OF TIME HAS PASSED, THERE IS A PERIOD OF RECOVERY (WHICH MAY OR MAY NOT BE 'NON FUNCTIONING').'

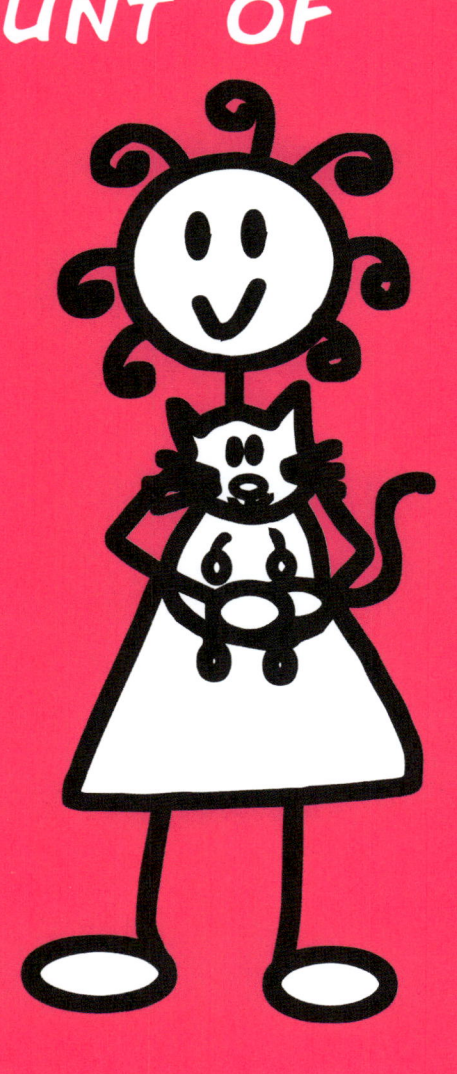

'I need to get back to routine. That is the most important thing to me and, when I'm out of routine, it plays on my mind so much that I can't focus on anything other than that ticking "routine clock."'

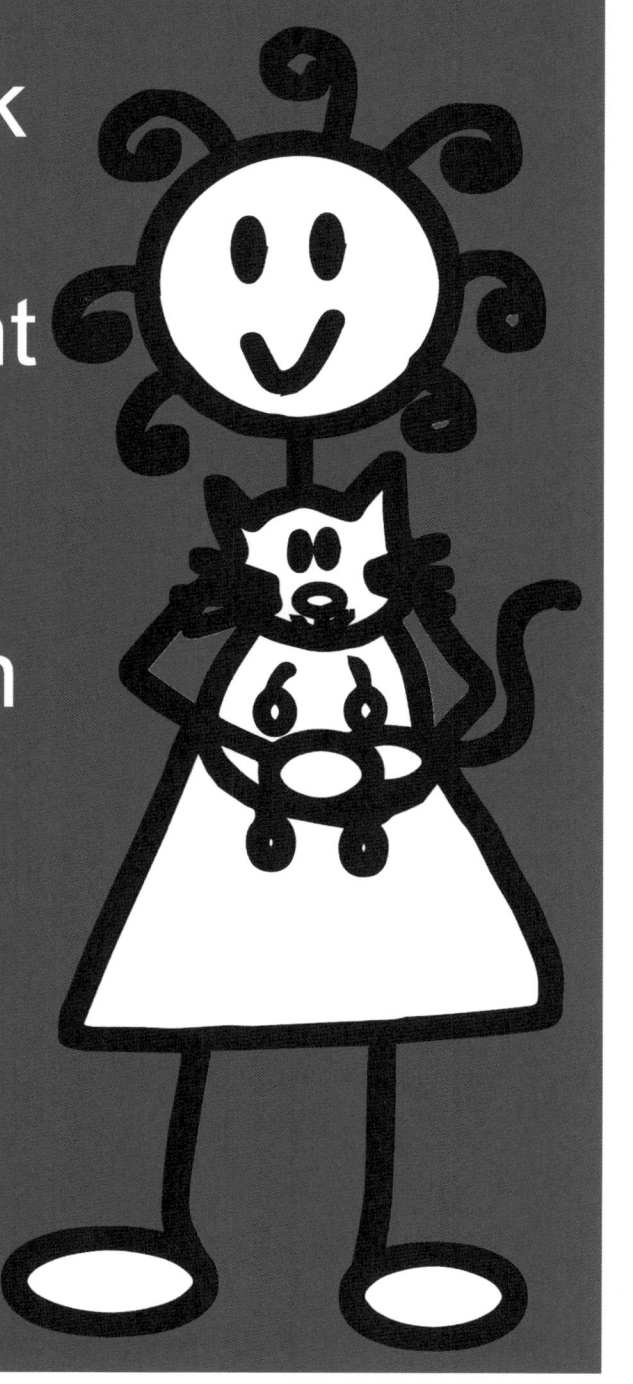

'When I am meeting someone somewhere, I will always be early because 1) I like to use the extra time to 'settle into' the new situation, and 2) my anxiety is always so high that I am not able to focus on doing any other tasks before the meeting anyway.'

'IT IS VERY HARD FOR ME TO COPE WITH MISTAKES IF FOR NO OTHER REASON THAN I DO NOT HAVE A PLAN B.'

'I might not conform to societal rules and "norms" but I still care deeply about how I come across to others and I would never want someone to consider me selfish, rude or unkind.'

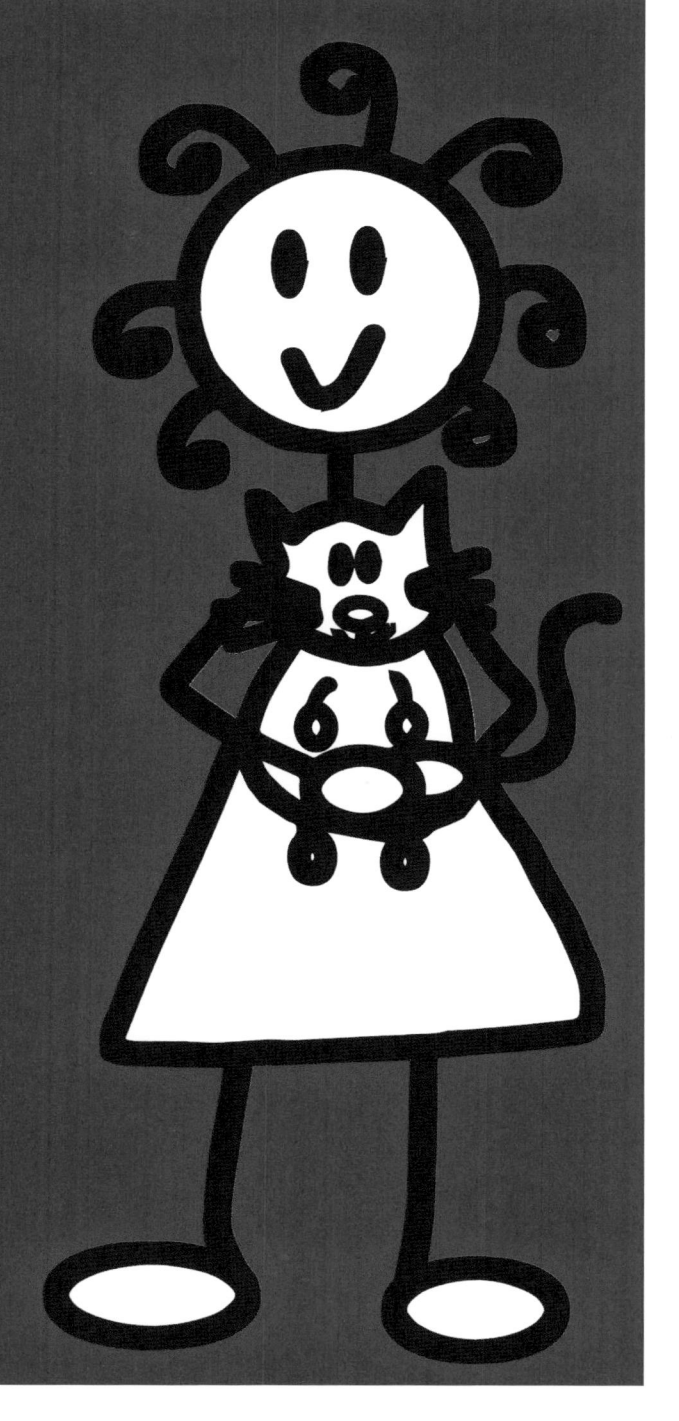

'I live in the present a lot, but that means I tend to 'forget' how angry or sad I really am/was. But then at some point I just end up having a complete meltdown. This then comes as a surprise to others, who thought I was fine.'

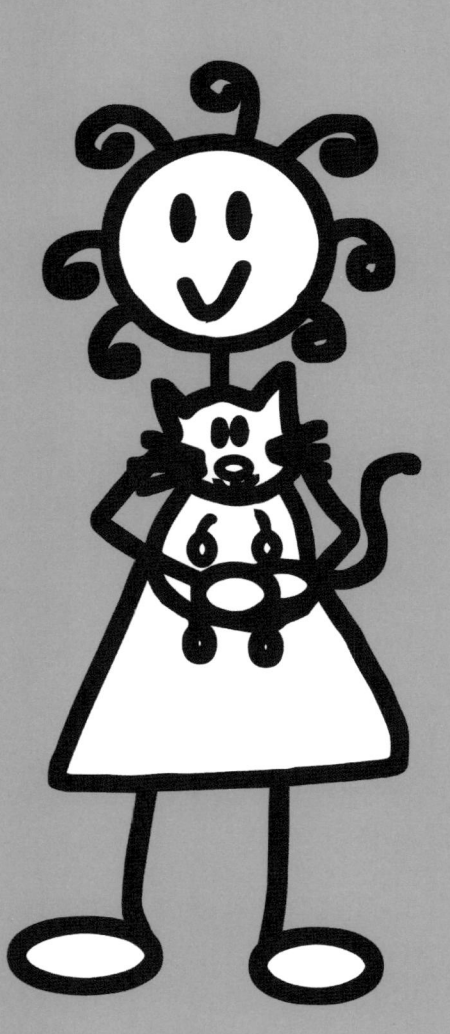

'When I talk about anxiety that is debilitating, I am not referring to visits to the doctor, taking exams, going to interviews, etc. ... I am talking about the anxiety I have just being in the presence of others, or when there are changes to my routine.'

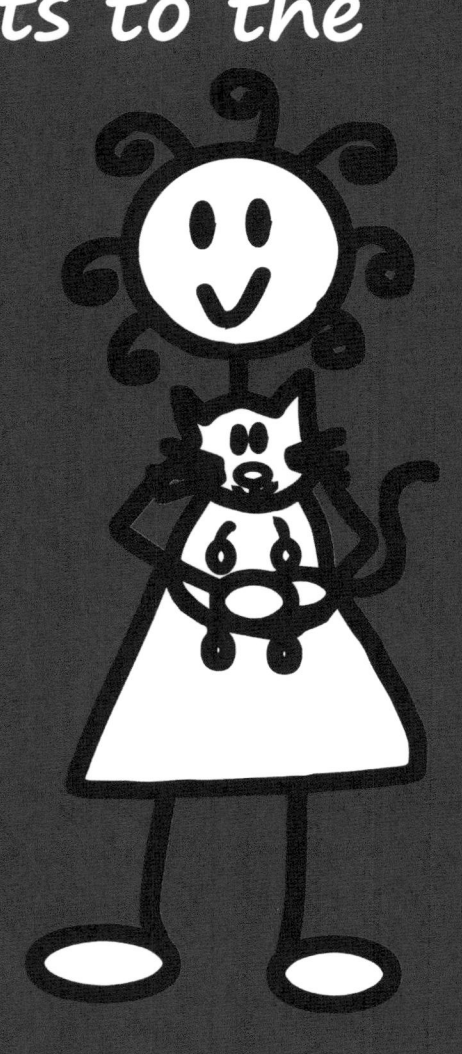

'As an introvert with ASD, I wish more people (especially extroverts) would understand that, just because they get their pleasure from being around others, it doesn't mean I do/will. I have "down days" like lots of people but, by choosing not to socialise, doesn't automatically mean I am making myself feel worse.'

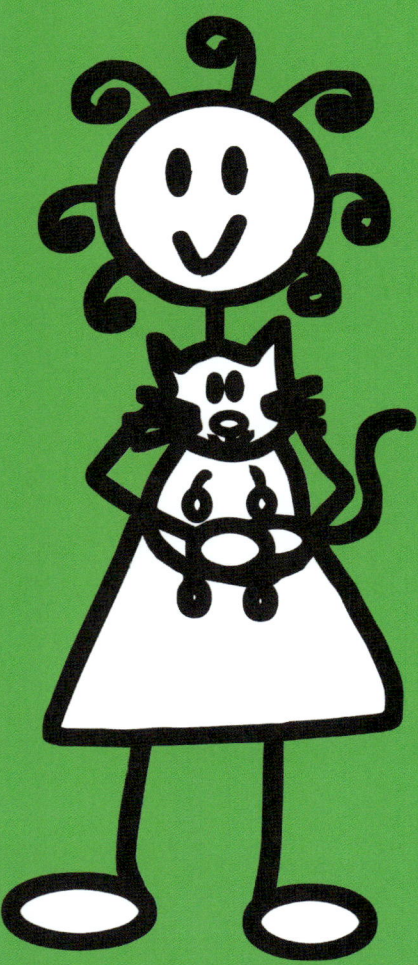

'When deciding on whether to meet someone, it's not about whether I am "free" or "busy." It's about my social energy levels; it is about how I am feeling on the day. And that is hard to plan for.'

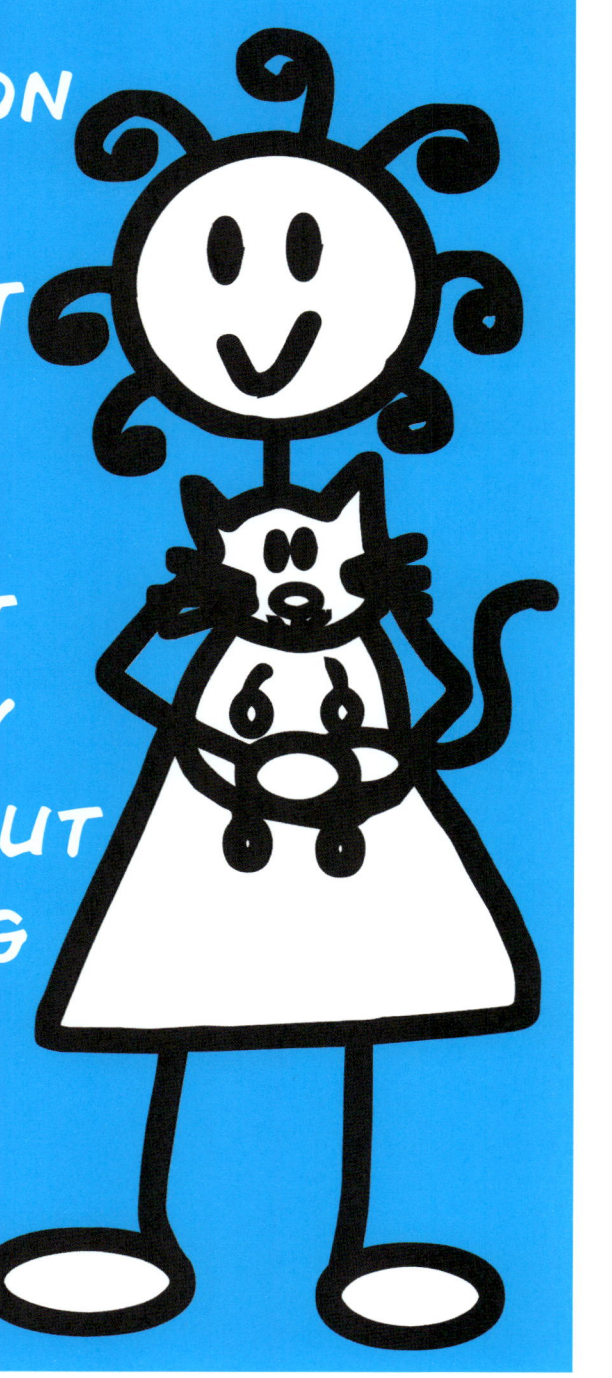

'I come across as young but not just because of how I look. It's also because of the way I dress, having body language that is always slightly 'off', the excitement I show for certain things, the things I talk about, and the memories, metaphors and analogies I refer to, the life experiences I've had (and not had).'

'It takes me a long, long time to adjust to changes. What I mean by this is, there will be a transition period of adjustment before thechange, and then a period of adjustment after the change. I feel very, very anxious and unsettled until a routine is re-established.'

'I can only really ever enjoy something if I have approached it in two main ways: 1) I need to know all the details of the event, e.g. start and end time, transport arrangements, meal times, free times, etc., and 2) I need to have planned for any contingencies that might change the event.'

'I am not overly anxious around strangers but, as soon as these strangers become acquaintances, that can all change, and I will start to feel very anxious around them.'

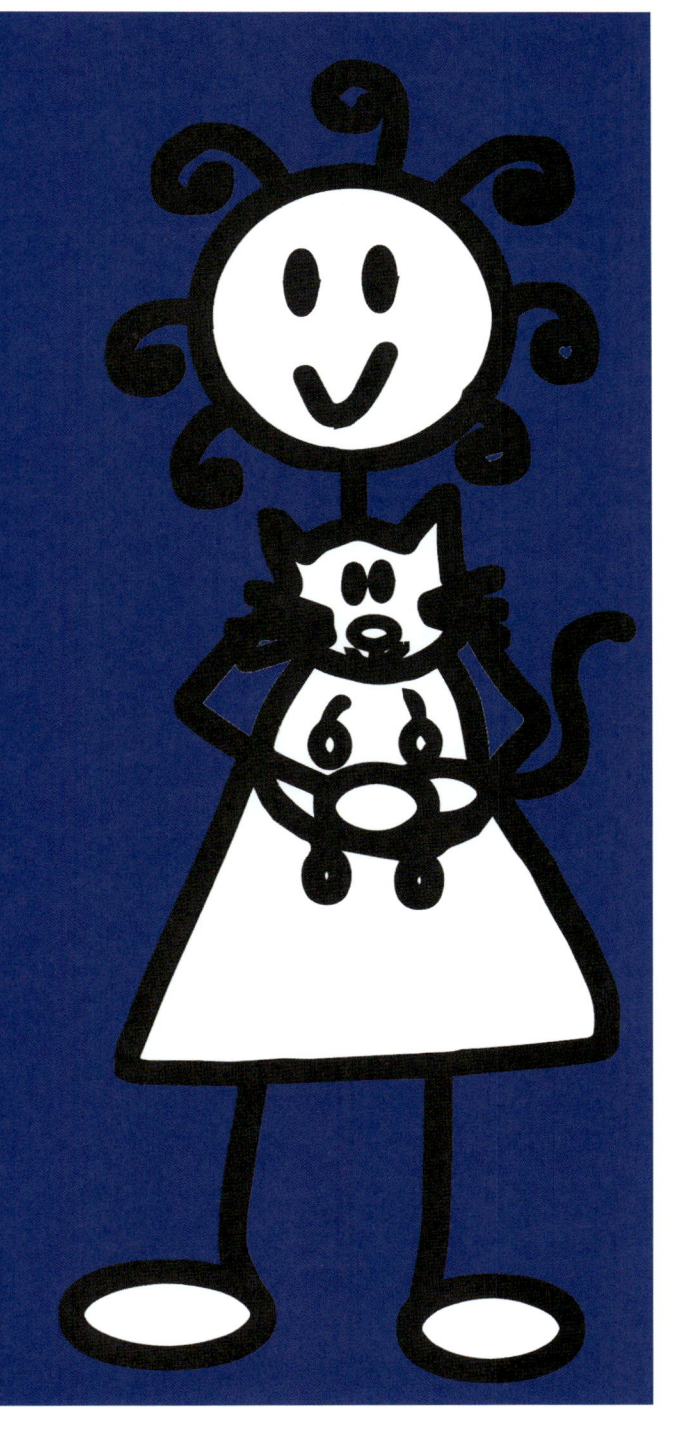

'I can detect by my senses (sight, smell, sound, etc.) what is going on around me a lot more quickly than most people.'

'Sequences are very important to me. I manage my day to day life using sequences, e.g. I do this first, then this and then this, etc.'

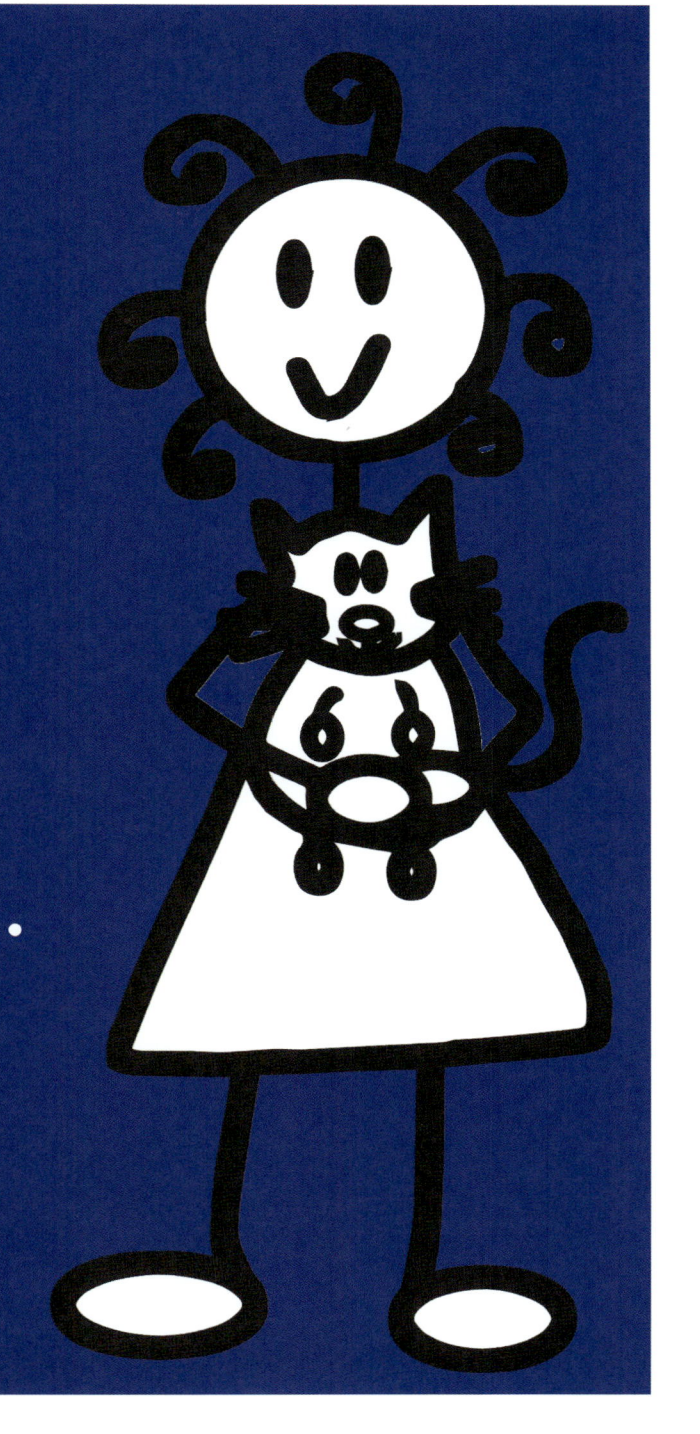

'For me, anxiety and sadness are closely linked. Confusion is always the first step, which leads to anxiety, which leads to hopelessness, which leads to sadness.'

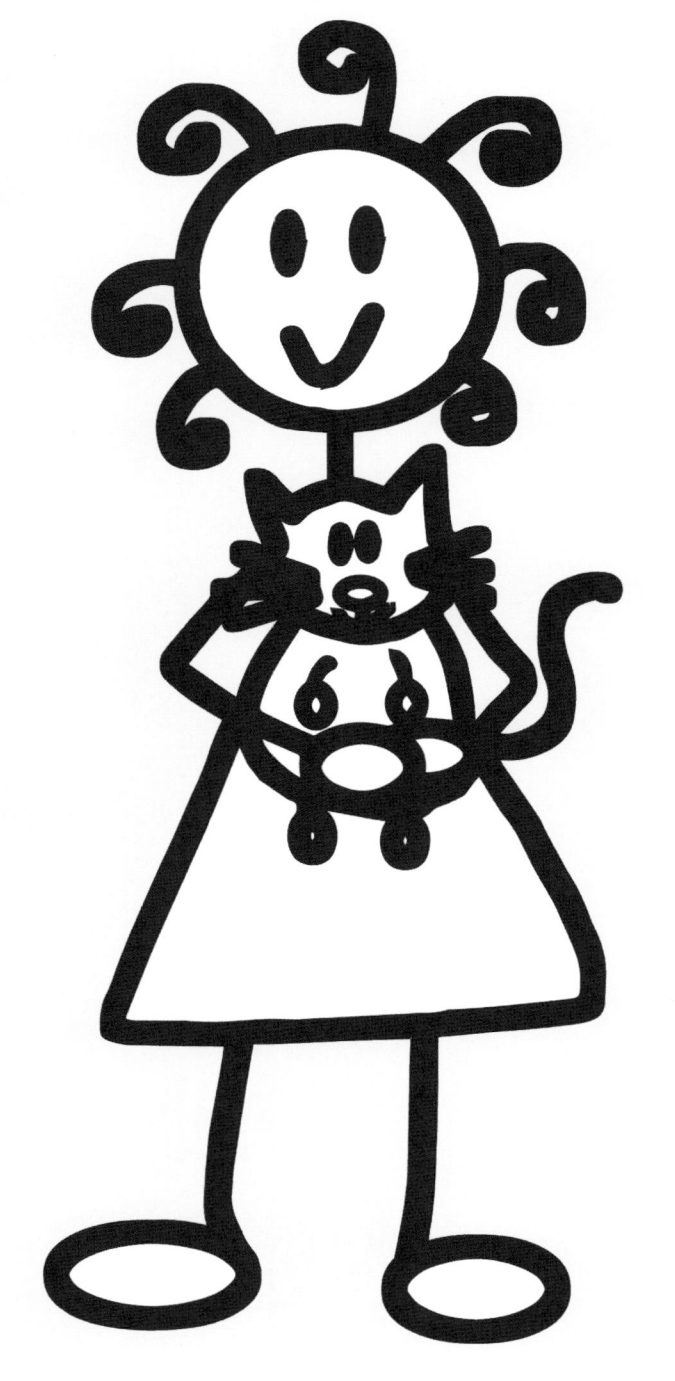

'As human beings, our experiences of things are all different. A "strong" smell or a "bright" light may not be strong or bright at all to someone else.'

'I experience fatigue on a daily basis. For every day that I am out of the house for any length of time, I get very fatigued by the end of the day. Even if I haven't 'done' much, just being out of my home, around people, in different environments, is exhausting.'

'For us, 'socialising' can be anything involving a social interaction - the 5 minutes in the playground before school starts, the vague but constant chit chat at work, bumping into an old friend in the street, etc. All of these things may as well be 'socialising' for us, because they involve social interactions, and we do not have the intuitive social skills or the ability/social "ease" that NTs have.'

'It astounds me how neurotypical people have the energy to do things in the evenings or at the weekends, even after - or despite - doing all their 'normal' things during the weekdays. For me, I just crash.'

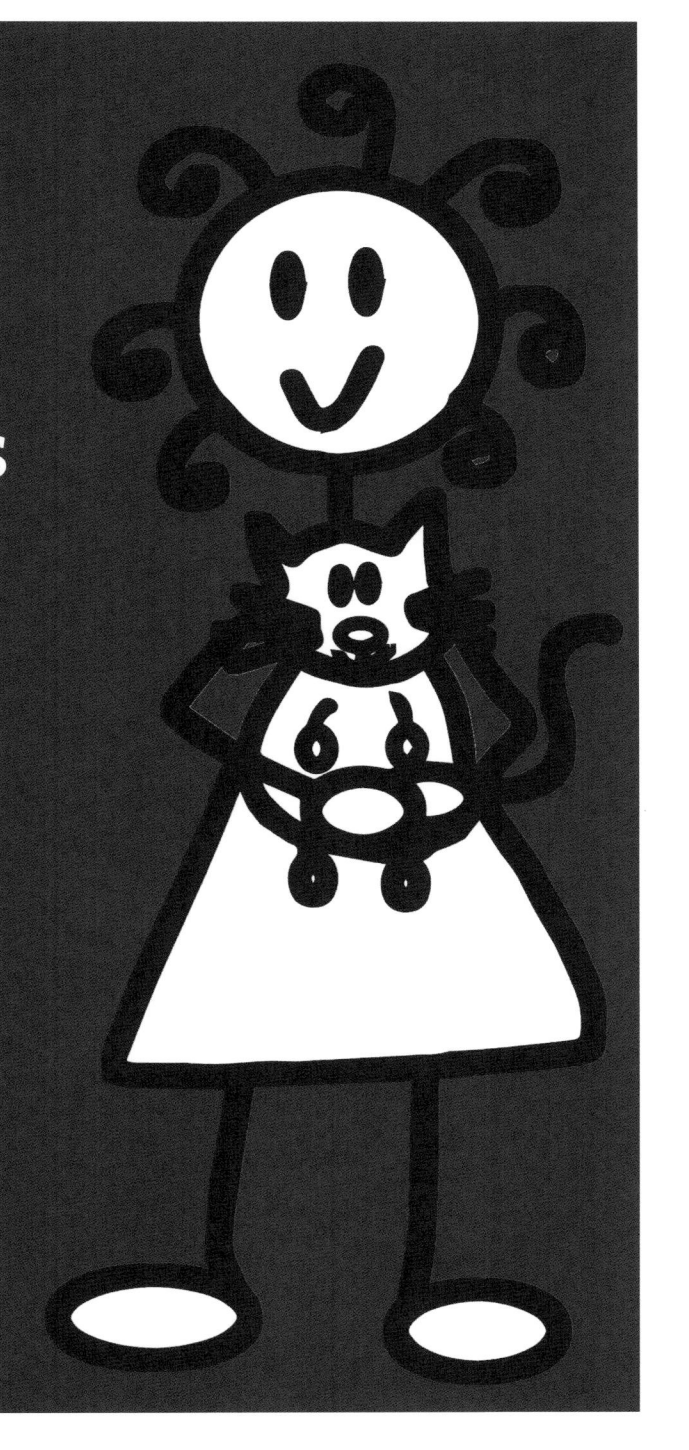

'On the outside, I come across as being a bit quirky but still quite capable and clever. It is a shock to some people when they find out I am quite severely disabled in lots of ways.'

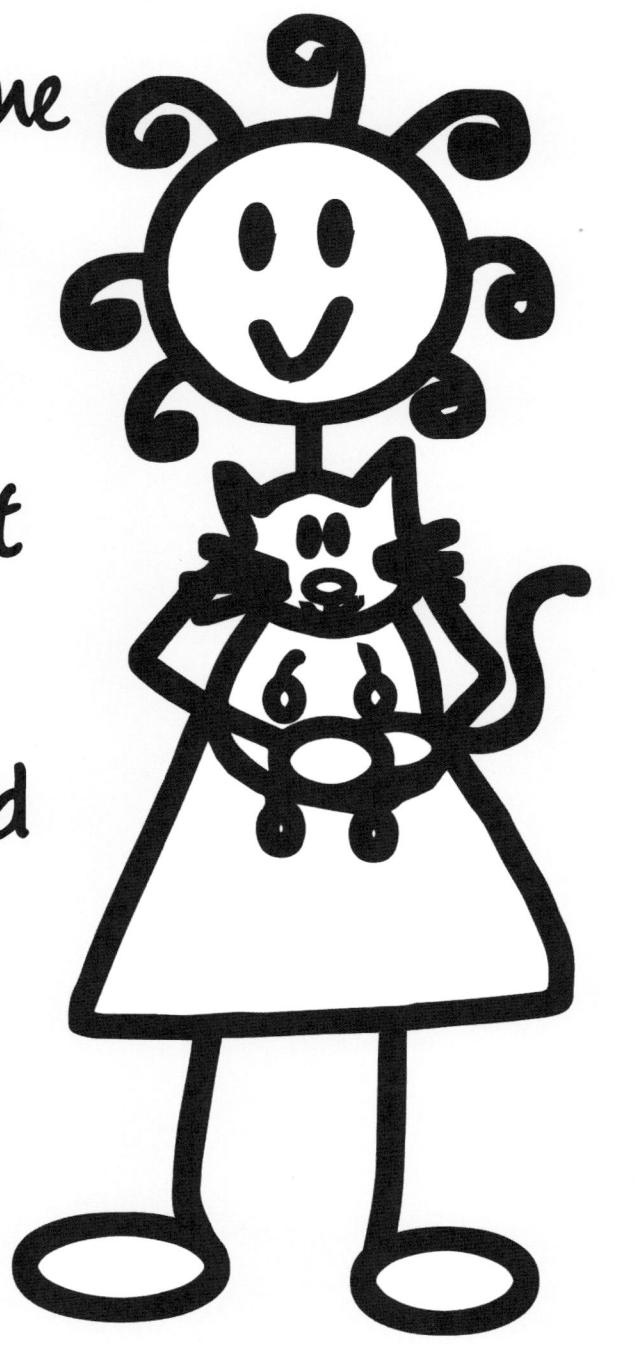

'I know very very clearly what I like and what I dislike. I don't even feel I have to try something to know whether or not I'm going to like it - the knowledge is already there. I am so content, most of the time, that I don't need to look for anything else more exciting to be doing.'

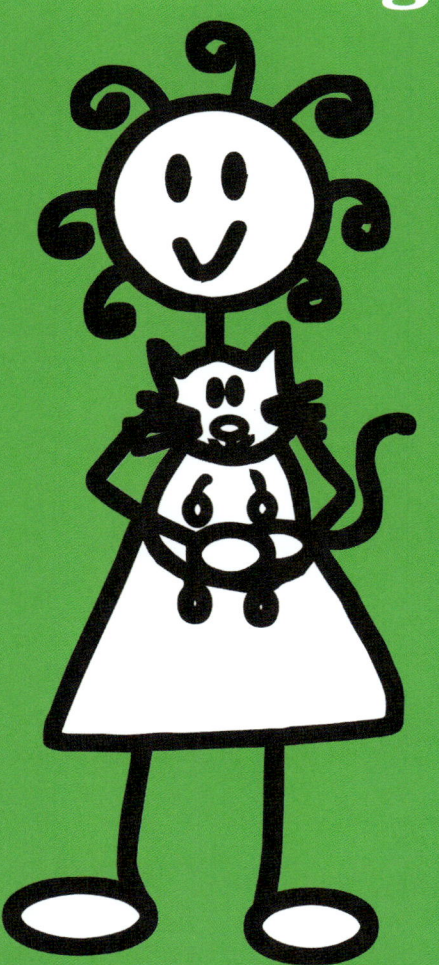

'My priorities in life are: my routine, my alone time, and my special interest.'

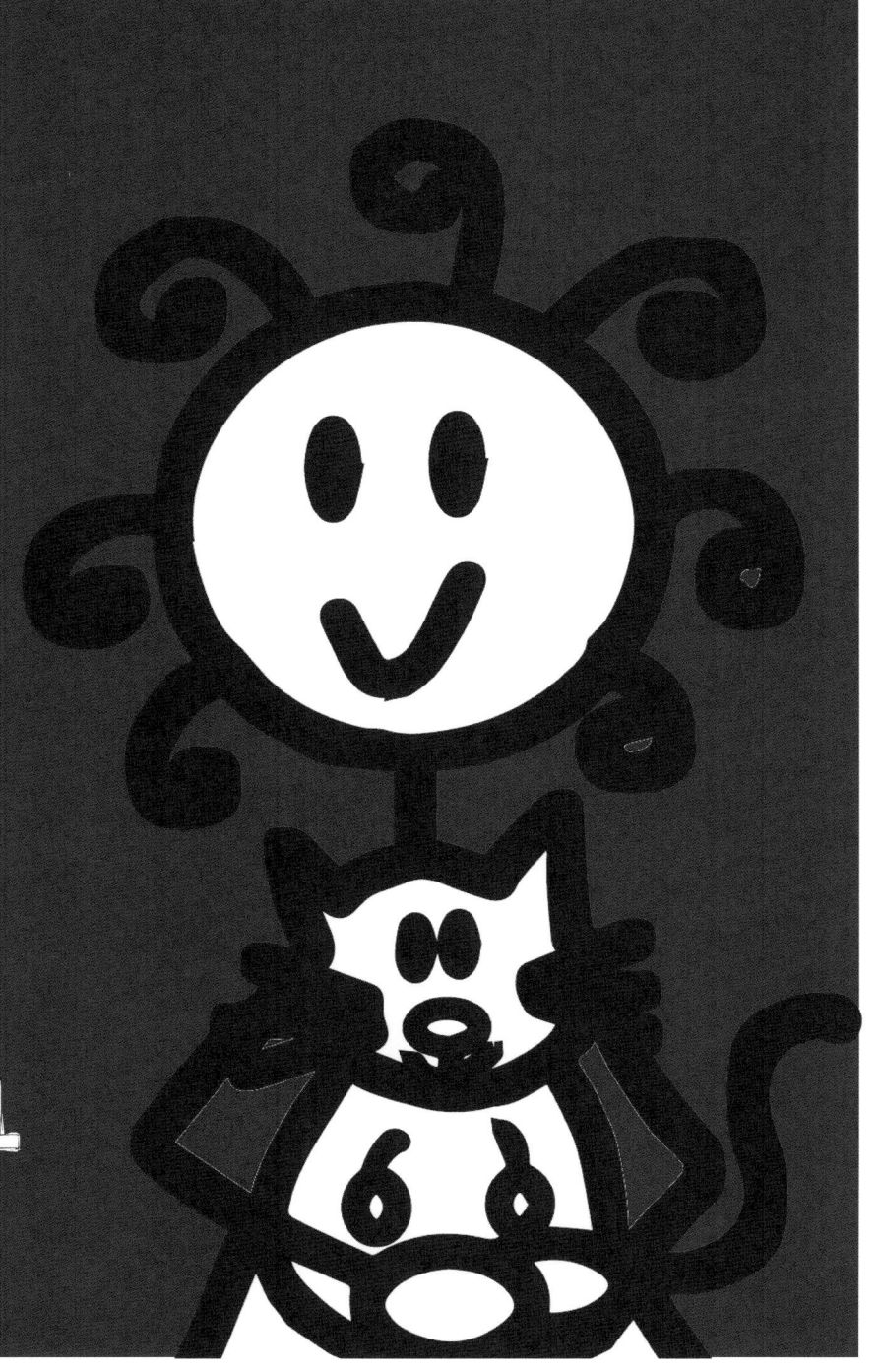

'Time is really, really important to me. Having tasks that are timed (start as well as end) is basically how my whole life is organised and how I manage my anxiety. Without timings, I feel incredibly anxious.'

'I have a lot of free time, but I can't - and don't - want to use it for socialising. I wish more people understood that.'

'Meeting up with someone isn't as straightforward as simply having a space in the diary. It all depends on social energy on the day, the tasks before and after the space, and careful consideration for the amount of social energy required for those tasks too.'

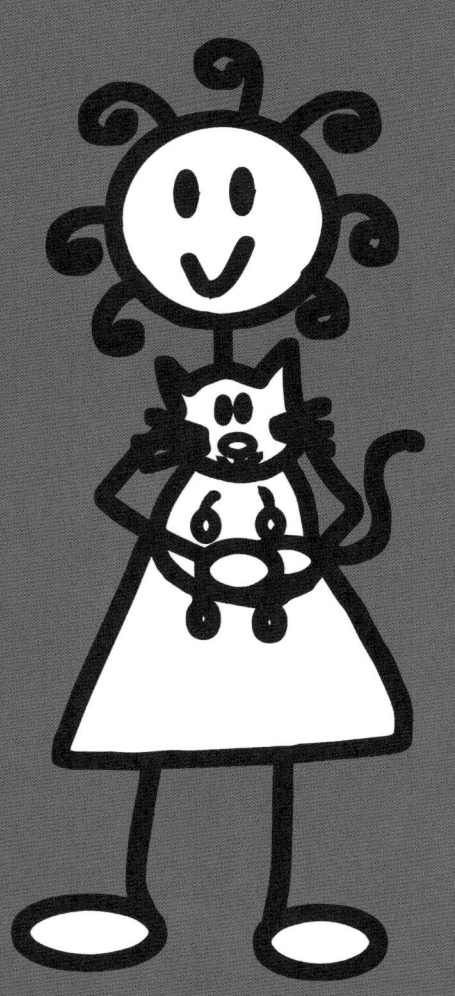

'I PREFER NOT TO BE TOO EMOTIONAL IN EITHER DIRECTION (GOOD OR BAD). IT EXHAUSTS ME TO FEEL THOSE EXTREMES, I ACTUALLY FEEL LIKE I CAN'T HANDLE THEM. I FEEL BEST WHEN I AM JUST CONTENT AND CALM.'

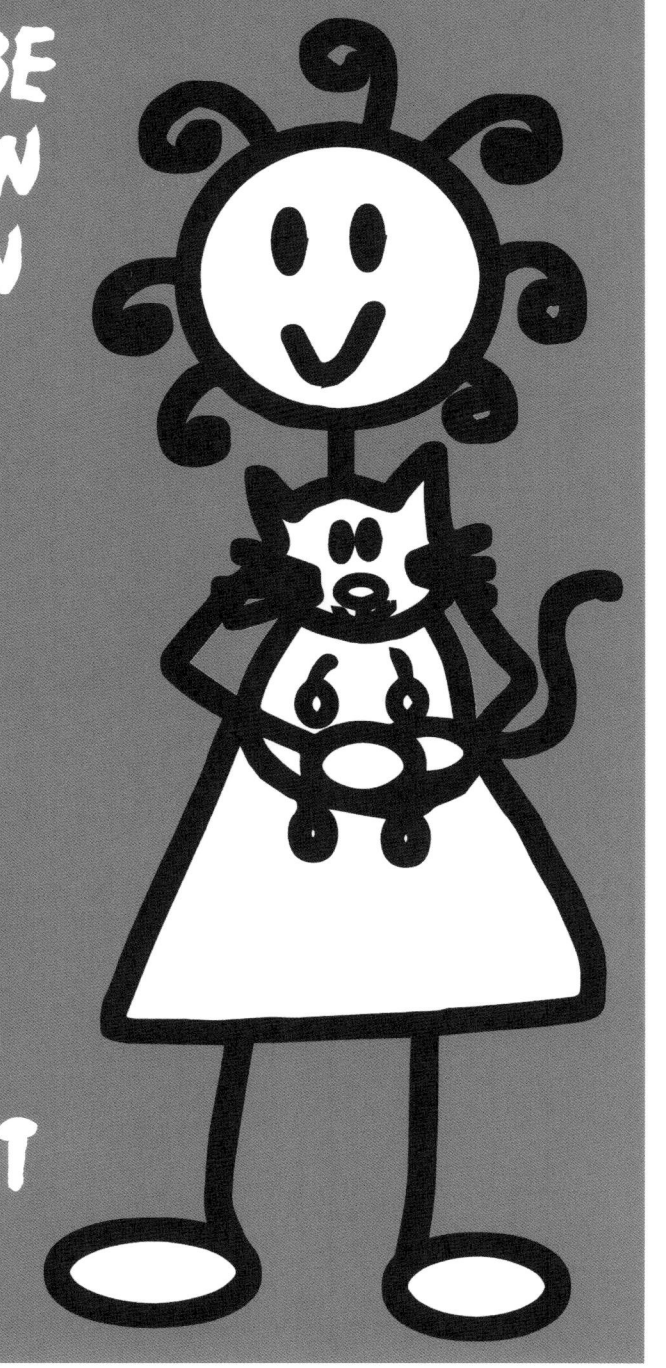

'I plan out everything step by step. Everything I do is a result of a lot of thinking! I don't rush into everything. Even if it appears I have done something recklessly, I've actually most likely been pondering it a long time.'

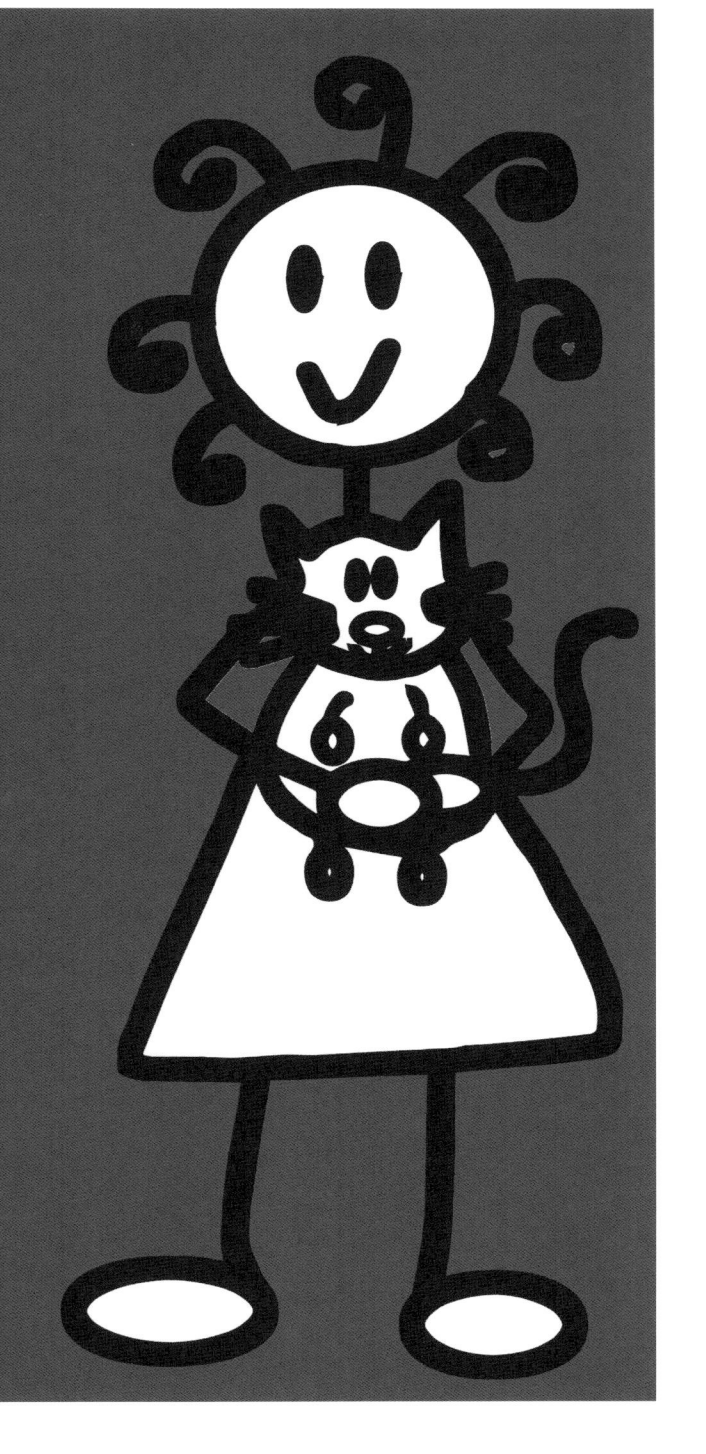

'I like to be up very early in the morning. At this time, the whole world is deserted; visitors are unlikely, phone calls are likely… Basically, at this time, any sort of social interaction is unlikely.'

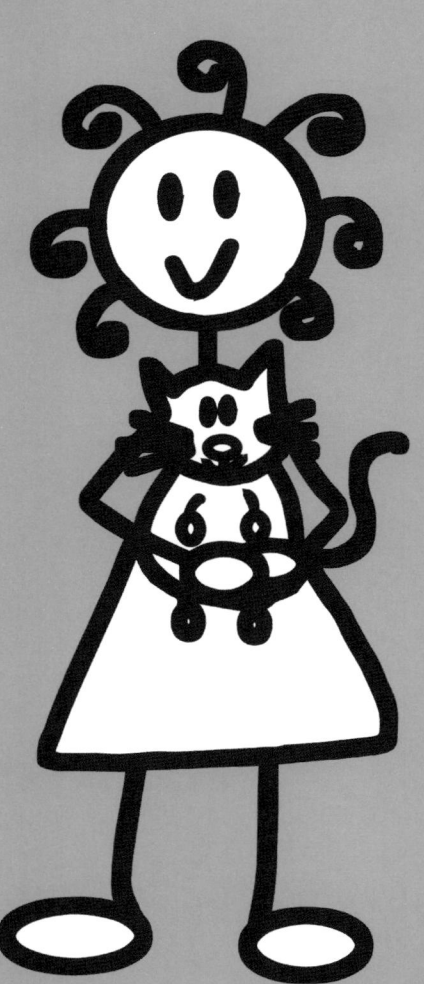

'The presence of another person still takes up my attention, even if we're not talking. Their presence is still often distracting.'

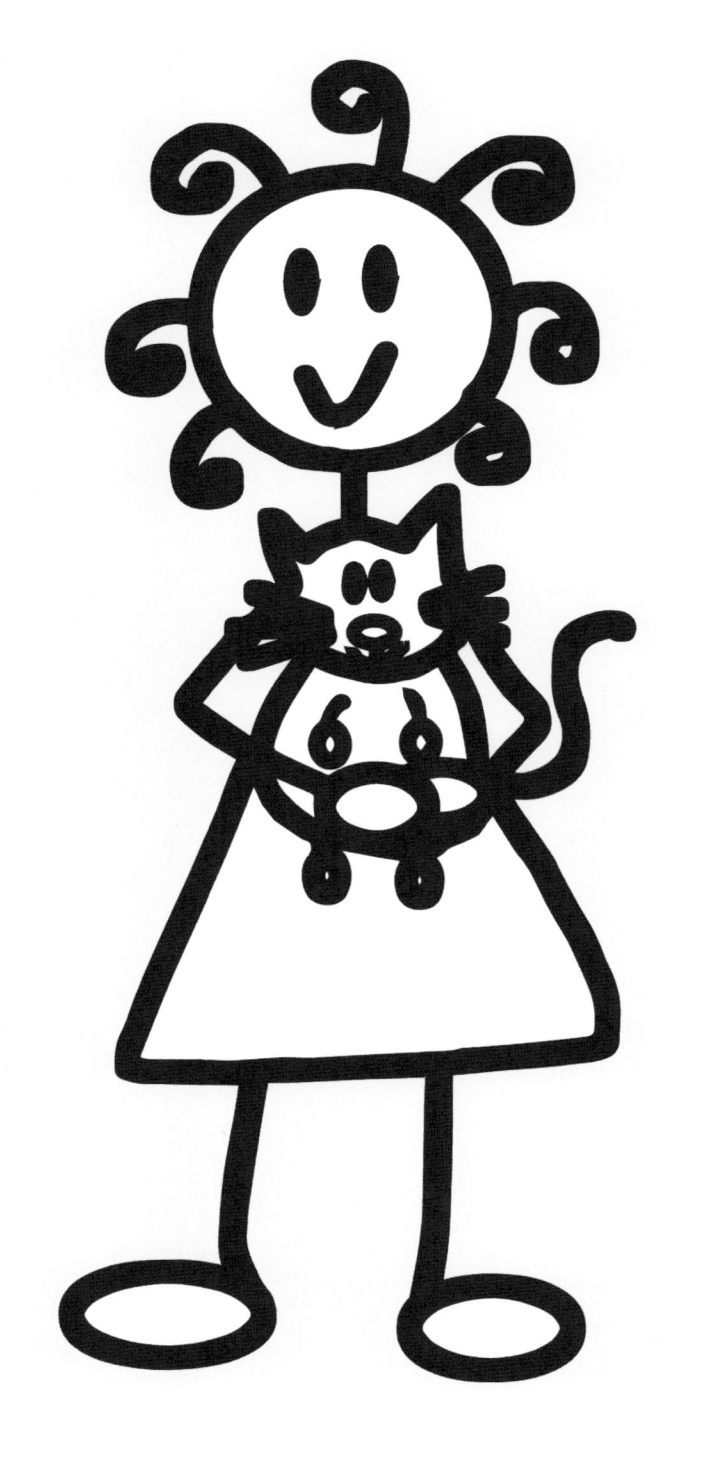

'WHEN YOU THINK AND SEE THINGS DIFFERENTLY, YOU ARE GOING TO ACT AND REACT TO THINGS DIFFERENTLY. THESE ACTIONS AND REACTIONS CAN APPEAR ODD OR SURPRISISING TO OTHERS BUT THEY'RE VERY NORMAL AND SENSICAL TO US.'

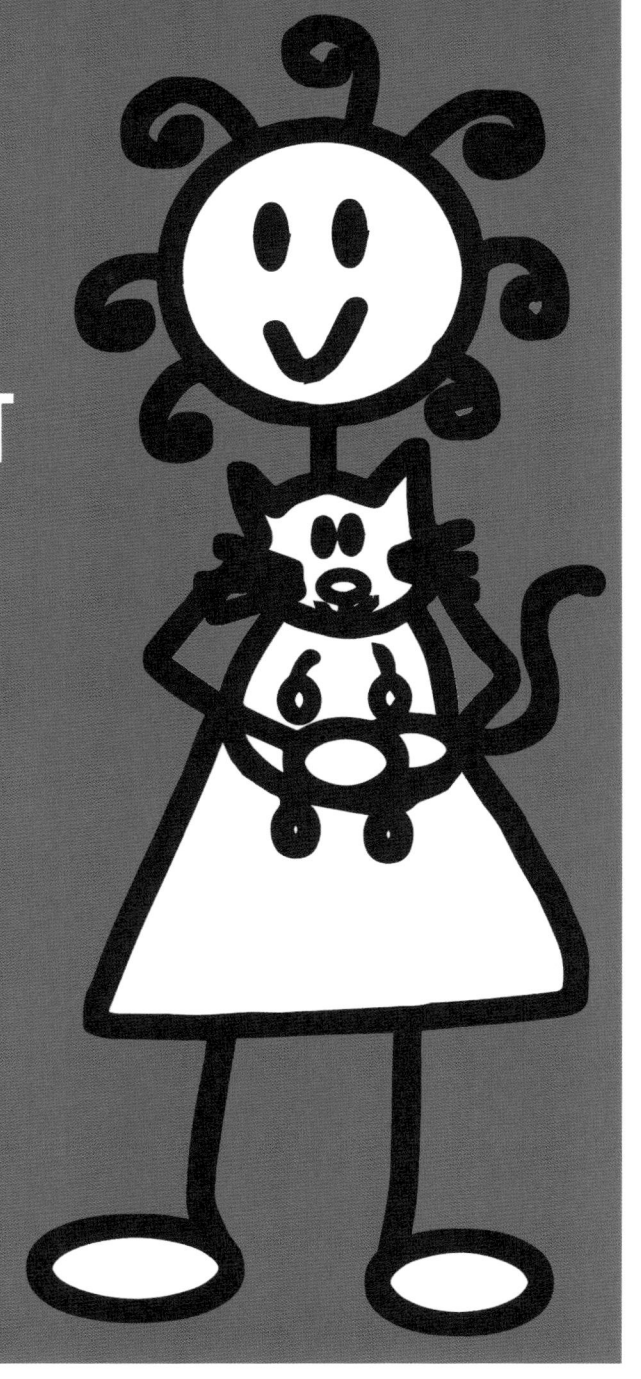

'I am very competent and adept in some areas of my life, but I still struggle with doing 'everyday things.' Often, when people see the clever, efficient, skillful things I can do they think I should be just as competent in other areas of my life. Then they can't understand why I'm not.'

'I am not the same person in the night time as I am during the day. In the day time, I use up all my social energy doing the 'normal' tasks of life and, by night time, there is no more left. You can somewhat expect me to function and do "things" during the day (in fact, you can even ask me to do things!), but, I will not be able to do those same things later on.'

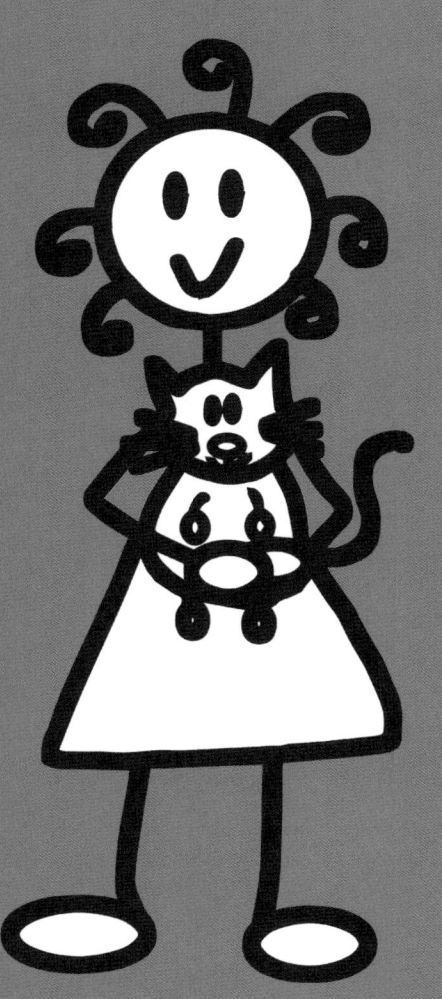

'A routine doesn't just mean the way the person plans their day, it can be the way they fold the laundry, the way they wash the dishes, the order in which they get dressed, etc.'

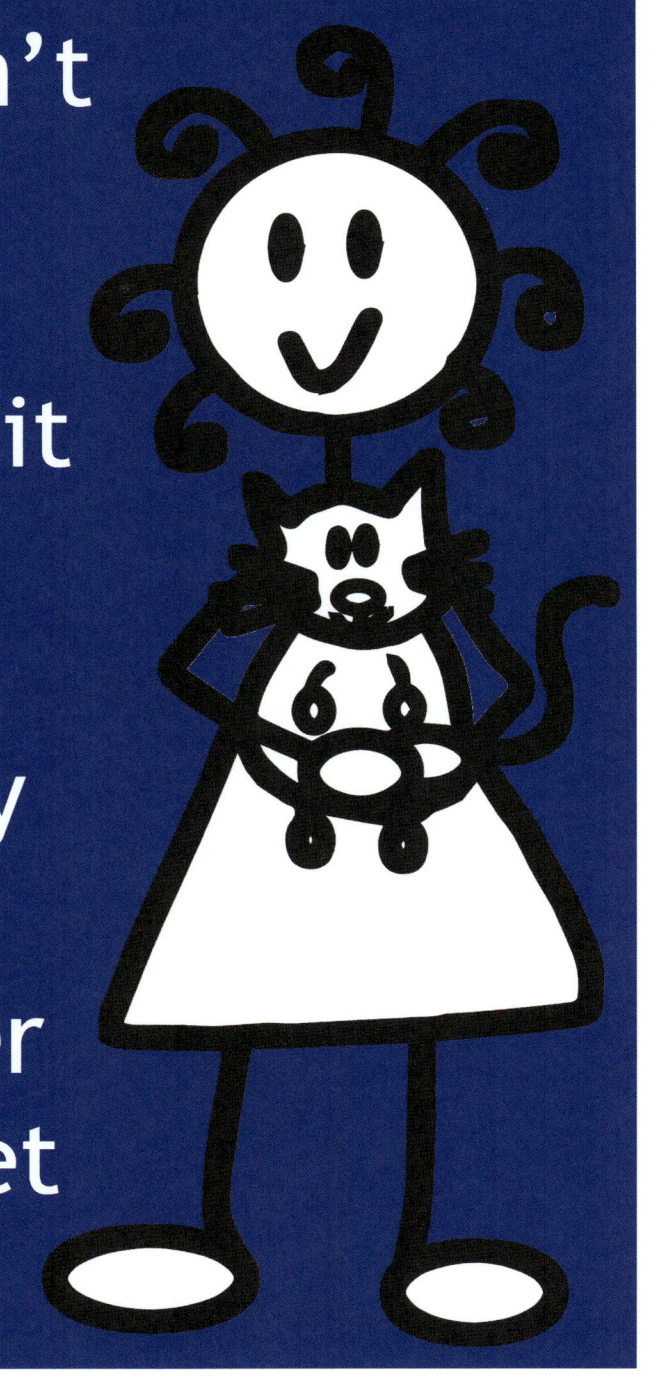

'It's very important for people with ASD to get the balance right between time spent with loved ones and time spent with acquaintances, classmates, colleagues, peers, etc. If too much time is spent with the latter, they will experience the glass jar feeling very strongly, which can lead to social anxiety and low mood.'

'I am highly dedicated. If I care about something, I will put in a lot of effort and stick at it, and the end result will be very high quality.'

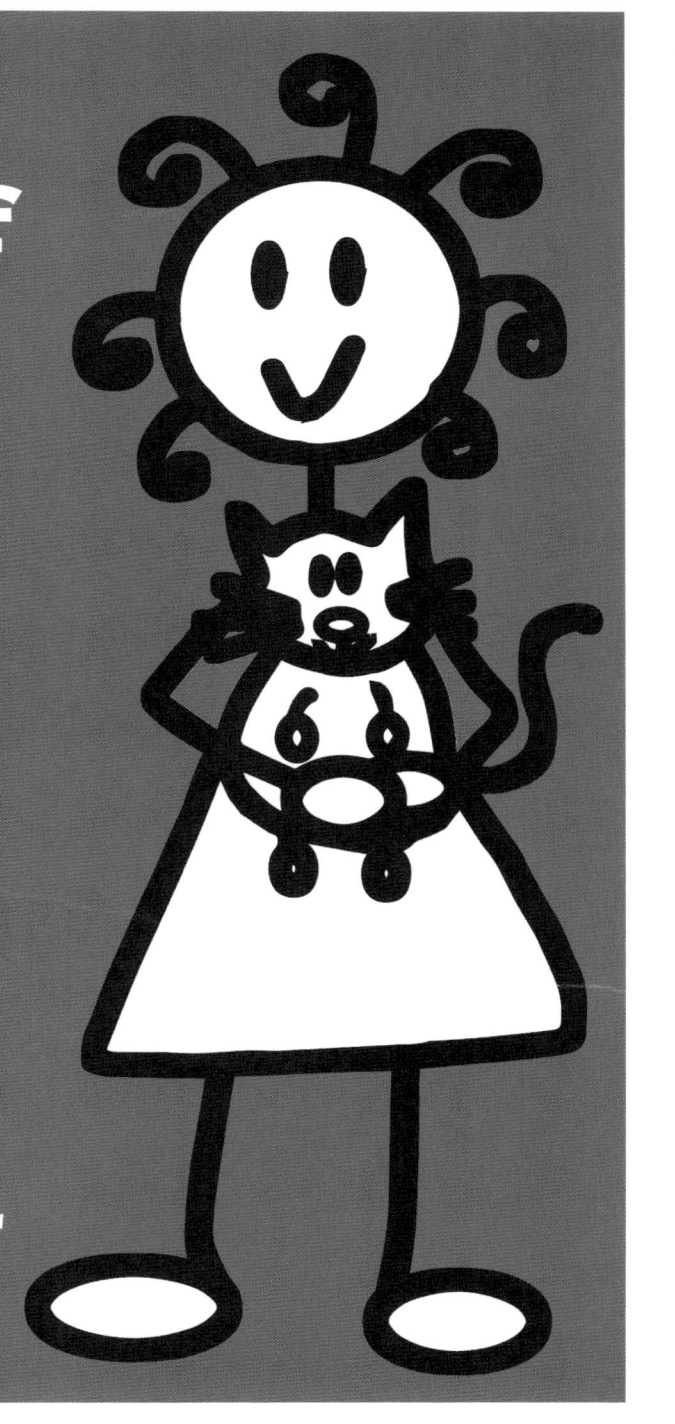

'I like other people just fine but I still need lots of of self-centering, alone time after social interactions, even after social interactions I have enjoyed.'

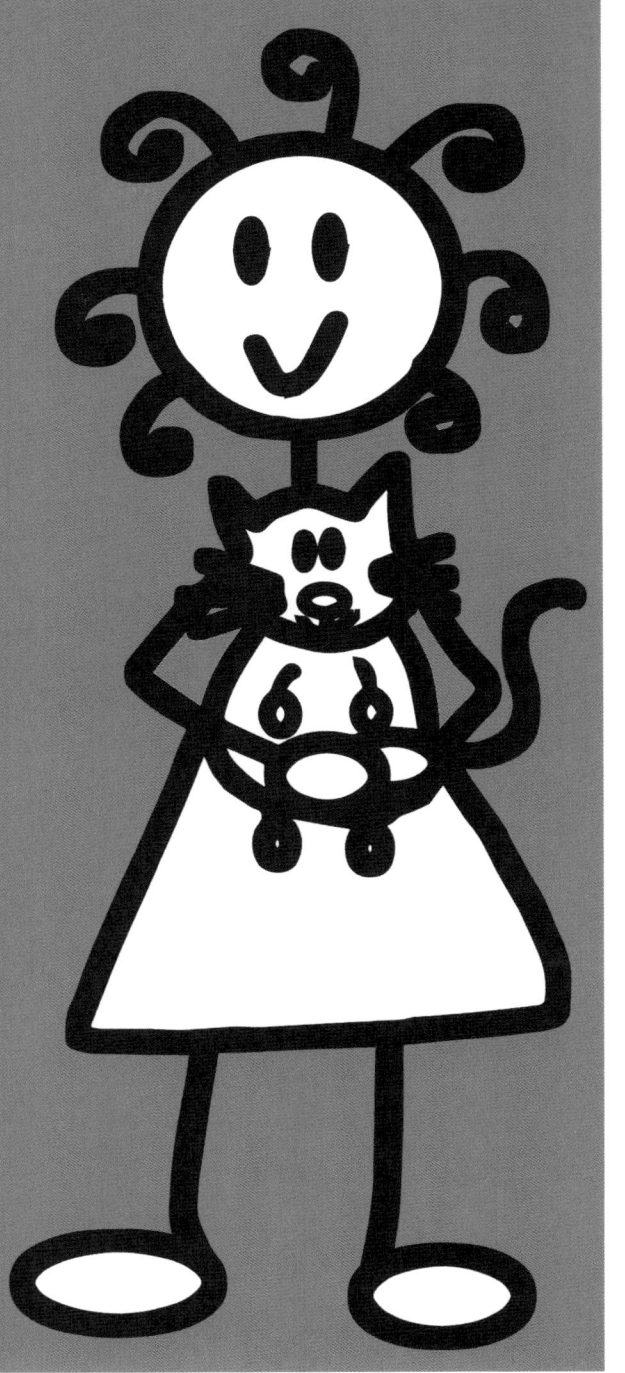

'Spending time around people (who are not like me) makes me feel incredibly alienated. Being reminded of the things other people do or the things they enjoy doing just emphasises my feelings of feeling different.'

'To me, right and wrong are so clear and distinguishable. It confuses and frustrates me when they are not to others.'

'I go about my life feeling pained, wondering why I get so upset over things that do not really bother others; wondering why something affects me so much more than others; wondering why can they get over something when I can't? Makes me feel very lonely and 'different' every single day.'

**For more memes,
visit www.facebook.com/
thegirlwiththecurlyhair**

Printed in Great Britain
by Amazon